Laís Lima
Aniclécio Lima
Talita da Silva

HPV and cervical cancer

Laís Lima
Aniclécio Lima
Talita da Silva

HPV and cervical cancer

How does this happen?

ScienciaScripts

Imprint

Any brand names and product names mentioned in this book are subject to trademark, brand or patent protection and are trademarks or registered trademarks of their respective holders. The use of brand names, product names, common names, trade names, product descriptions etc. even without a particular marking in this work is in no way to be construed to mean that such names may be regarded as unrestricted in respect of trademark and brand protection legislation and could thus be used by anyone.

Cover image: www.ingimage.com

This book is a translation from the original published under ISBN 978-3-639-74603-7.

Publisher:
Sciencia Scripts
is a trademark of
Dodo Books Indian Ocean Ltd. and OmniScriptum S.R.L publishing group

120 High Road, East Finchley, London, N2 9ED, United Kingdom
Str. Armeneasca 28/1, office 1, Chisinau MD-2012, Republic of Moldova, Europe
Printed at: see last page
ISBN: 978-620-6-47828-7

HPV AND CERVICAL CANCER

Lais Rocha Lima

Aniclecio Mendes Lima

Talita Pereira Lima da Silva

New Academic Editions

Thanks

We thank God for the gift of knowledge and for guiding us along this professional path so that we can contribute our knowledge to science and health;

To our family members for always supporting and encouraging our choices;

To all the people involved in putting this book together, thank you for your hard work, dedication and commitment;

Thank you to everyone!

TABLE OF CONTENTS

1

ANATOMY OF THE FEMALE REPRODUCTIVE SYSTEM

Lais Rocha Lima

Aniclécio Mendes Lima

The female reproductive system has delimited internal and external organs that are attached to the pelvic floor and are connected by a canal called the vagina, in which anatomical and structural integrity is related to the proper functioning of the genitourinary system. The pelvic cavity is of great importance in protecting the external genitalia, as well as providing important functions such as mating and parturition.

The female reproductive organs undergo significant functional and structural changes on a monthly basis, and these changes do not occur to make women's lives meaningless, but are fundamental at the beginning and during the gestational period. If pregnancy doesn't occur, the endometrial lining will flake off and shed, reaching the vagina as menstrual blood. These activities take place under the action of hormones released by the female sex organs in accordance with the endocrine system. Female sex hormones play an important role in sexual maturation.

STRUCTURE OF THE FEMALE REPRODUCTIVE SYSTEM

The internal organs of the female reproductive system are located inside the pelvis and comprise the ovaries, fallopian tubes, uterus and vagina. The external organs are superficial to the urogenital diaphragm and are located below the pubic arch and consist of the labial formations, vestibule of the vulva, erectile organs and adnexal glands.

The internal organs of the female reproductive system are located in the lower part of the abdominal cavity. These include the ovaries, the fallopian tubes, the uterus and the vagina. The external genitalia are made up of the vulva and the pudendum. The mammary glands are also considered part of the female reproductive system. We will now look at some specific structural and functional characteristics of each structure.

OVARIOS

The ovaries or female gonads are women's reproductive glands, located in the lower region of the abdominal cavity, one on each side of the uterus and below the fallopian tubes, and held in this position by various ligaments, These include the broad ligament, which also supports the fallopian tubes, the uterus and the vagina, as well as the tubo-ovarian ligament, the utero-ovarian ligament and the mesovarium, which is a double peritoneal fold that joins the hilum of the organ to the posterior leaflet of the broad ligament.

The female gonads have a shape similar to an almond, and their location can vary according to the emptying and filling of nearby structures, such as the urinary bladder and the intestine. They are made up of an internal part, called the medullary portion, which is responsible for nutrition and ovarian endocrine activity, and a peripheral portion called the cortical portion, where folliculogenesis takes place.

The ovaries are covered by the peritoneum, which is a serous membrane made up of simple epithelial cells called the germinal epithelium. Underneath the germinal epithelium is a layer of fibrous connective tissue, the albuginea tunic, which is responsible for the whitish color of the ovary and underneath this tunic there is a cortical region, in which the ovarian follicles that contain the oocytes predominate. In this context, the follicles are located in the connective tissue of the cortical region, and after maturation they are released by the ovaries and captured by the fimbriae of the fallopian tubes, where they will be stored for the arrival of the spermatozoon, so that fertilization can take place.

The ovaries are supplied by the ovarian arteries which arise from the abdominal aorta, and these blood vessels travel through the suspensory ligaments to reach the gonads. Venous drainage is carried out by the pampiniform plexus and innervation is carried out by the ovarian nerve plexus, which receives fibers from the aortic, renal and hypogastric plexuses (superior and inferior), as well as the pelvic splanchnic nerves.

UTERINE TUBES

The fallopian tubes are two flexible muscular organs between 7cm and 14cm long that extend towards the walls of the pelvis, where they fold over the ovaries. They are responsible for capturing the female gamete released by the ovary in the peritoneal cavity and leading it to the uterus.

The fallopian tubes are divided into 4 parts: the intramural part, the isthmus of the tube, the ampulla of the tube and the infundibulum. The intramural part is the section of the tube that is located in the wall of the uterus, and at the beginning of this tube there is an opening called the uterine ostium of the tube, which establishes its communication with the uterine cavity. The isthmus is the least calibrous segment and corresponds to the medial third of the fallopian tube and dilates from the ampulla to the uterus. The ampulla is the volatile portion of the tube and is considered to be the region in which the process of fertilization of the ovum by the sperm takes place. The distal end of the tube is the infundibulum, which has irregular edges and folds, the fimbriae, and opens spontaneously into the cavity of the peritoneum through the ostium of the fallopian tube and settles over the ovary.

The fallopian tubes are made up of three concentric layers of tissue: the mucous layer; the serous layer, formed by a visceral layer of peritoneum; and the muscular layer of smooth muscle. The mucous layer has many parallel longitudinal folds called tubal folds, which are reduced in the segments of the tube closest to the uterus, and this layer is formed by a simple epithelium with ciliated and secretory cells and composed of loose connective tissue. The muscular tunic, represented by smooth muscle fibers, is divided into internal and external and is made up of loose connective tissue between them and a layer of connective tissue and mesothelium, called the serosa, which helps the ova migrate towards the uterus and provides the tube with peristaltic movements.

The uterine tubes are vascularized by the uterine and ovarian arteries. The venous drainage of this organ is carried out by the tubes which drain into the uterine venous plexuses. Sympathetic innervation comes from the superior hypogastric plexus via the hypogastric nerve, while parasympathetic innervation comes from the pelvic splanchnic nerves and the vagus nerve.

ÙTERO

It is a hollow fibromuscular organ, median and flattened anteroposteriorly, which arises from the center of the perineum into the pelvic cavity, whose function is to store the fertilized ovum during its development and expel it when it reaches maturity, providing the maintenance of the human species. The uterus is located in the center of the small pelvis between the bladder and the rectum and below the intestinal wings above the vagina, into which it is inserted.

The uterus, in its normal state, is about 7 cm long and 5 cm wide with an inverted pear shape, the upper region of which is called the body. Below the body, the uterus narrows to form the isthmus and when it connects to the vagina, it forms the cervix. The dome-shaped portion of the uterine body above and between the points of the fallopian tubes is called the fundus and the opening of the uterus into the vagina is called the ostium of the uterus.

The wall of the uterus is made up of three overlapping layers, from the outside in: serous (perimetrium), muscular (myometrium) and mucous (endometrium). The serous layer represented by the visceral peritoneum covers the visceral region, as well as the intestinal region of the organ at the level of the lateral borders. The subserosal tunic is characterized by a sheet of connective tissue located between the serous tunic and the muscular tunic. The muscular tunic or myometrium is made up of a layer of smooth muscle fibers distributed from periphery to depth in 3 planes: longitudinal, plexiform and circular. The endometrium is made up of a superficial layer and a thin layer lining the entire uterine cavity, which undergoes intense developmental changes during the course of the menstrual cycle.

The uterus is held in place by three ligaments: the broad ligament of the uterus, the round ligament of the uterus and the uterosacral ligament. These ligaments don't hold the uterus firmly in place, but instead provide limited movement. In this context, the muscles and membranes that surround the pelvic floor are the main supports of the uterus, since these muscles are attached to a tendon posterior to the opening of the vagina, called the perineal tendon center.

The uterus is supplied by the uterine arteries (branches of the internal iliac artery) and accessorily by the uterine branches of the ovarian arteries (branches of the abdominal aorta). Venous blood drainage is carried out via the uterine venous plexus into the internal iliac vein. As far as the innervation of this organ is concerned, it is mainly carried out by the uterinovaginal nerves. The vessels and nerves run through the lateral ligaments (broad ligament of the uterus), a wide duplication of the peritoneum connecting the lateral wall of the uterus with the pelvic wall.

VAGINA

The vagina is a membranous muscular canal that extends from the cervix to the vestibule of the vulva, flattened anteroposteriorly and oblate inferiorly and anteriorly, forming a 70° angle with the horizontal plane, with the exception of its distal third, which is almost vertical. The vagina is made up of two walls, one anterior and one posterior, which remain attached along their length, forming a virtual cavity. This organ is shaped like a cylindrical tube in the upper segment to enclose the vaginal portion of the uterine cervix, which is flattened transversely to conform to the female pudendum inferiorly.

The anterior portion of the vagina is short and the posterior portion is longer, with the upper part of the vaginal canal surrounding the cervix, forming a recess, the fornix of the vagina. The long portion of the recess, situated dorsally to the cervix, is called the posterior fornix or posterior part of the fornix.

It is the woman's copulating organ and is made up of transverse folds and longitudinal columns. Its main support comes from the communication between the levator ani muscles and the tissue that joins it bilaterally to the walls of the pelvis. In addition, the cardinal ligaments, endopelvic fascia, perineal body and pubovesicocervical fascia also provide support and fixation.

The entrance to the vagina is protected by a circular membrane, the hymen, which is responsible for partially obstructing the vulva-vaginal duct, and this hymen usually breaks during the first sexual intercourse. The vaginal canal has Bartholin's glands on its sides, whose function is to secrete a mucous-like substance that lubricates the vagina, facilitating penetration by the penis during sexual intercourse, when stimulated by the parasympathetic nervous system.

The vagina is irrigated in its upper part by descending or cervical branches of the uterine artery, in the middle part and in the lower part by the vaginal artery and branches of the female pudendum. The venous drainage of the vagina is carried out by the vaginal veins, which discharge into the internal iliac veins. This organ is innervated by the inferior hypogastric plexus, the uterovaginal plexus and at the distal end by the pudendal nerve via the deep perineal nerve.

EXTERNAL ORGANS OF THE FEMALE REPRODUCTIVE SYSTEM

The vulva or female pudendum consists of a set of external genital organs comprising labial formations (pubic mound, large and small labia), vestibule or interlabial space, erectile organs (clitoris and vestibular bulbs) and adnexal glands (major and minor vestibular glands). The external genitalia are devoid of numerous sensory and tactile nerve endings, as well as Meissner's and Pacini's muscles, which contribute to the physiology of sexual stimulation.

The pubic mound is a prominence made up of fibrous tissue and covered in hair that begins to appear after puberty. It serves to protect the pubic bone, which is located in front of the pubic symphysis, i.e. in the triangle of the upper base.

The labia majora are folds of skin made up of adipose tissue and a thin layer of smooth muscle. Their inner surface is histologically similar in structure to the labia minora, while their outer surface is covered with thick hair and skin. The labia majora extend from the pubis to the perineum, helping to protect the opening of the vagina and urethra from infectious agents such as fungi and bacteria. Inside, there are sebaceous and sweat glands.

The labia minora are thin folds made up of vaginal mucosa and connective tissue that are located inside the labia majora. The stratified sidewalk epithelium that covers them has a thin layer of keratinized cells on the surface. They are very sensitive areas that increase in volume when a woman is sexually aroused, because they are abundantly innervated and vascularized. They demarcate the vestibule region, where the openings of the vagina and urethra are located. It also has a large number of sweat and sebaceous glands, but no hair. Furthermore, in the upper region, they form the prepuce of the clitoris, while in the lower portion they form the frenulum or posterior commissure.

The vestibule is the elongated space between the labia minora, the upper part of which is formed by the clitoris and the base by the frenulum. This organ has several orifices: for the urethra, the vagina, the major and minor vestibular glands. Inside the vestibule are the urethral meatus, the vaginal introitus and the Bartholin's glands, which are responsible for vaginal lubrication.

The clitoris is the erectile organ located at the top of the vulva, near the urethra and the junction of the labia minora, made up of spongy tissue called the corpus cavernosum. The visible parts of the clitoris are relatively small and correspond to the prepuce and glans, while the rest of the organ extends inside the body. It also has numerous nerve endings which are crucial to female sexual pleasure.

The vestibular bulbs are two small, even, elongated masses of erectile tissue, which are located next to the ostia of the vagina and urethra. The anterior ends of the bulbs form two thin cords that join near the glans of the clitoris, while the ends communicate with the larger vestibular glands.

The larger vestibular glands are located on each side of the lower opening of the vagina, below the vestibular bulbs and have an ovular aspect with a diameter of 0.5 to 0.8 cm. These major glands are responsible for secreting mucus which lubricates the distal part of the vagina.

The minor vestibular glands vary in number and their tiny ducts open in the vestibule of the vagina, between the ostium of the urethra and that of the vagina, and are responsible for producing secretion before and during intercourse in order to make the structures moist and facilitate sexual intercourse. These minor glands include mucous glands of two types according to their location: the paraurethral glands, which are located below the urethra, and the periurethral glands, which are located above the urethra.

The external genitalia receive their arterial supply from the internal and external pudendal arteries, which are respectively branches of the internal iliac arteries and the femoral arteries. Venous drainage is provided by the internal and external pudendal veins. The anterior region of the vulva is innervated by the ilioinguinal nerves and the genitofemoral nerves. The posterior portion is innervated by the pudendal nerve and the posterior cutaneous nerve of the thigh. The vestibular bulb and clitoris are innervated by the utero-vaginal nerve plexus.

MAMMARY GLANDS

The mammary gland is a paired organ, located on the anterior wall of the thorax, resting on the pectoralis major muscle and extending from the second to the sixth rib in the vertical plane from the sternum to the anterior axillary line in the horizontal plane. Each mammary gland is made up of 15 to 20 gland lobules and alveolar tubules, with a skin-covered prominence located superficially to the pectoralis major muscles. In addition, below each mammary gland there is a nipple surrounded by a circular areola. The nipple as well as the areola is pigmented and has capillary beds situated just below its surface.

The mammary gland is made up of two different tissues: the parenchyma and the stroma. The glandular parenchyma has morphological units (adenomers) responsible for milk secretion, while the glandular stroma is the tissue that contains blood capillaries, myoepithelial cells and reticular fibers, and is defined as intraparenchymal interstitial connective tissue.

Breast growth, differentiation and lactation involve the processes of mammogenesis, lactogenesis and galactopoesis. Mammogenesis can be understood as the growth and development of the mammary gland; lactogenesis is the way in which breast alveolar cells acquire the ability to secrete milk and galactopoiesis refers to the maintenance of milk secretion.

The histological structure of the mammary glands varies according to sex, age and physiological state, and their development begins after puberty, when they are exposed to cyclical stimulation by estrogens and progesterone. In addition, breast enlargement at puberty can also result from the accumulation of adipose and connective tissue, as well as some growth and branching of the galactophorous ducts.

The mammary gland is vascularized by the superior thoracic, lateral thoracic, thoracic-acromial, internal thoracic and posterior intercostal arteries, the first three of which are collateral branches from the axillary artery. The innervation of this organ comes from sympathetic nerves that reach the gland with the arteries that irrigate it; cutaneous and lateral branches of the third to sixth intercostal nerves; supra-clavicular branches of the cervical plexus and thoracic branches of the brachial plexus.

REFERENCES

AIRES, M. M. (org.). **Physiology**. 4. ed. Rio de Janeiro: Guanabara Koogan. 2012.

ALBERTS, B; BRAY, D; LEWIS, J. **Molecular Biology of the Cell**. 5. ed. Porto Alegre: Artmed, 2009.

BERNARDES, Antonio. Surgical anatomy of the female genital tract. **Manual of Gynecology**. **Permanyer Portugal**, 2011.

BERNARDES, Antonio. Anatomy of the female breast. **Manual of Gynecology**, v. 2, n. 12, p. 12-24, 2011.

BERNE, R. M. et al. **Physiology**. 6. ed. Rio de Janeiro: Elsevier, 2009.

CAMPBELL, N. A., et al. **Biology**. 8. ed. Porto Alegre: Artmed, 2010.

GUYTON, A.C; HALL, J. E. **Treatise on Medical Physiology**. 12. ed. Rio de Janeiro: Elsevier, 2011.

JUNQUEIRA, L. C; CARNEIRO, J. **Female reproductive system**. **Basic histology**. Editora Guanabara, Rio de Janeiro, Brazil, p. 335-355, 1990.

2

VIRUS

Lais Rocha Lima

Paulo Sérgio da Paz Silva Filho

The Human Papillomavirus (HPV) is known as a circular double-stranded DNA virus with a length of 7,900 kilobases, an icosahedral shape, non-enveloped, with 72 capsomeres. Papilloma Viruses are members of the Papovaviridae family and infect the epithelium of some animals, including reptiles, birds and mammals, as well as humans.

There are more than 200 types of Papilloma Virus, which are described by DNA sequences. Of these, 100 types have already been described as affecting humans and around 50 types that act on the mucosa of the genital tract have already been identified. The virus is classified according to the species of natural host and subclassified into types according to the nucleotide sequences of the DNA.

The virus is characterized by its small size, about 55 nm in diameter, and by being non-enveloped. Its genome is a double-stranded DNA molecule with around 8,000 paired bases, containing three regions: The distal or L region, where it has two genes - L1 and L2 - coding for the capsids of the virus proteins, the proximal or E region which acts by coding for the proteins present in viral replication and transcription control called E1 and E2 and the main genes that become E6, E7 and E5, as well as the long control region (LCR), linked to various sites that have nuclear, viral and disseminator sequencing transcription factors.

The LCR region is about 10% of the viral genome and contains gene regulatory elements such as promoters and transcriptional regulatory elements. The early *open reading frames* (ORFs) are six in number: E6, E7, E1, E2, E4 and E5 and they code for proteins that regulate the viral cycle, with E6 and E7 being the main oncoproteins, while (L1 and L2) are known as the late ORFs and code for the structural proteins of the viral capsid. The early proteins are expressed in cells in the early stages of cell differentiation and act as follows: E1 is involved in the replication of the viral genome, E2 acts in the adjustment of gene expression, cell cycle and apoptosis of the host cell, E4 is involved in the promotion of the keratin network by keratinocytes, E5 is involved in immune modulation, as well as the control of cell growth and differentiation, E6 and E7 stimulate cell proliferation.

HPV genomes are seen in the nucleus of cells infected with the virus, and infectious viral particles can be isolated in this region. In the cervix, in some low-grade lesions and in most high-grade lesions, HPV genomes are detected integrated into the chromosomes, and this integration is the fundamental point of oncogenic cell modification. HPV DNA integration deregulates the expression of E6 and E7, which interact with tumor suppressor genes p53 and RB proteins, respectively.

For the circular genome to be integrated into the host cell's DNA, it must be linearized by breaking the viral DNA between the E1 and L1 regions, resulting in the rupture or loss of the E2 gene, which is found in the most serious lesions, such as "in situ" and invasive carcinoma. Once HPVs have been integrated into the cell genome, they begin to encode the E6 and E7 oncoproteins which promote the malignant process. The host cell has the tumor suppressor genes RB and TP53. The RB gene is the main regulator of the cell cycle and the TP53 gene is called the "guardian of the genome", as it has the purpose of supervising that all the genes are integrated.

There are more than 150 types of HPV, 40 of which are found in the anogenital tract. The viruses are classified according to their risk, which can be high or low, depending on the epidemiological risk. Low-risk viruses are generally detected in vulvo-genital condylomas and high-risk viruses are associated with cervical cancer. Fifteen types of high-risk virus have been classified, including types 16, 18, 31, 33, 35, 39, 45, 51, 52, 56 and 58, while types 26, 53 and 66 are also considered probable high-risk types. The low-risk types are: 6, 11, 40, 42, 43, 44, 54, 61, 70, 72, 81 and types 34, 57 and 83 were, however, considered to be of undetermined risk.

Viruses are considered to be variants of the same type, so they are genotyped and not serotyped. The most commonly found in molecular laboratory tests and cervical or anal biopsy reports are 16 and 18, which are present in 70% of cervical cancers. Women with HPVs 16 and 18 have an increased risk of developing cervical cancer compared to those with other types. And genotypes 6 and 11, found in 90% of genital condylomas, are considered non-oncogenic. These present as individual or overlapping warts

Both oncogenic and non-oncogenic types of HPV can cause low-grade squamous intraepithelial lesions (LSIL) or cervical intraepithelial neoplasia (CIN 1) of the uterine cervix, which may or may not lead to the development of cervical cancer. HPVs 6 and 11 most often only cause infection and result in cell death. They cause the majority of genital warts in both men and women. HPVs 16 and 18, on the other hand, instead of leading to cell death, induce cell immortalization, thus enabling the oncogenic process. These are responsible for around 50% and 20% of all cases of cervical cancer in the world, respectively.

Some researchers have concluded that the incidence of high-risk HPV infections is higher than that of low-risk infections. HPV type 16 is the most dominant in genital tract infections, the most common in invasive cervical carcinoma and responsible for up to 66% of cases, followed by types 18 (15%), 45 (9%) and 31 (6%). The combination of these four types can account for up to 80% of cases.

In addition, HPV type 16 is the most prevalent in almost all parts of the world and the most persistent, lasting 12 months or more, while infections with other HPV types last 6-8 months. Thus, women with HPV types 16 and 18 have a higher risk of developing cervical cancer than those with other types.

REFERENCES

ANGELIM, J. L. C. **The hpv virus and cervical cancer**. Final course work. Universidade Paulista, Recife, 2014.

ILARDI, G. et al. Evaluation of HPV virus transcriptional status in a case of nasosinusal carcinoma. **International journal of molecular sciences** , v. 19, n. 3, p. 883, 2018.

HUBER, B. et al. L2-based chimeric virus-like particle (VLP) vaccines targeting cutaneous human papillomavirus (HPV). **PloSum** , v. 12, n. 1, p. e0169533, 2017.

YOUNG, D. et al. Increase in head and neck cancer in younger patients due to human papillomavirus (HPV). **Oncologia oral** , v. 51, n. 8, p. 727-730, 2015.

LAWSON, J.S; SALMONS, B. E; GLENN, W.K. Oncogenic viruses and breast cancer: mouse mammary tumor virus (MMTV), bovine leukemia virus (BLV), human papilloma virus (hpv) and epstein-barr virus (EBV). **Frontiers in oncology** , v. 8, p. 1, 2018.

LIMA, M. D. A. **Non-synonymous point mutations and their influence on the three-dimensional structure of the human papillomavirus (HPV) L1 protein**. Master's thesis. FUNDAÇÂO OSWALDO CRUZ, Recife, 2017.

LIMA, J. G. S;SILVA, R. B. F. HPV: The importance of cytopathologic examination in the detection of premalignant and malignant lesions of the cervix and anal canal. 2017.

LIRA, E.C. **Co-infection of human papillomavirus and chlamydiatrachomatis in women with normal and altered cytology.**Master's thesis. Federal University of Amazonas. Manaus. 2010.

NAKAGAWA, J. T. T; SCHIRMER, J; BARBIERI, M. Virus HPV and cervical cancer. **Revista Brasileira de Enfermagem**, v. 63, n. 2, p. 307-311, 2010.

PANTHAM, G. et al. Evaluation of the incidence of esophageal squamous cell papilloma and the presence of high-risk human papilloma virus. **Diseases of the esophagus: official journal of the International Society for Diseases of the Esophagus**, v. 30, n. 1, p. 1-5, 2017.

3

HISTORY

Lais Rocha Lima

Talita de Arêa Santos

In the first century of the Christian era, Martialis, a famous Roman satirical poet of Hispanic origin, in his *Epigrammata Medicae Philosophicae,* referred metaphorically to condylomata acuminata, genital warts, in a poem quoted by J. D Oriel in the chapter *Genital Warts in the book Diseases in the Homosexual Male,* organized by M. W. Aldler (1988). Apparently, genital warts were quite common and Greek and Roman physicians were the first to observe the sexual transmission of these lesions. At that time, the focus was on describing the signs, symptoms and treatment of diseases, but their causes were still unknown.

Genital warts were later considered to be a sexually transmitted disease related to homosexuality and lack of cleanliness in the genital organs, having been mentioned in various Greek and Roman writings, and were listed by Hunter in 1786 as a manifestation of slphilis. Its real viral etiology was uncovered by Strauss, Shaw, Bunting et al. in 1949 through electron microscopy on layers of warts. The apparent sexual infectivity of the verrucous lesions led Barret, Silbart and Mcginley in 1954 to think that it might be a sexually transmitted disease. As interest in the subject grew, various studies and experiments were developed and added to over the years, helping to identify various types and subtypes of the virus in the study of prevalent cases.

It was only at the end of the 19th century that the infectious nature of warts was recorded. In 1891, Joseph F. Payne, in London, published a classic article: *On the contagiousness of common warts, in* which he presented the development, by self-inoculation, of warts on his own thumb after having scraped the surface of a child's warty lesion. Shortly afterwards, in 1894, in independent studies, C. Licht and Gaston Variot also demonstrated the infectious nature of these lesions, resulting in the appearance of warts in volunteers inoculated experimentally with macerates of verrucous tissue.

The appearance of genital warts was associated with sexual promiscuity and seen as potentially infectious in the view of the Greeks and Romans. Since the 1920s, there have been reports of warty lesions on the skin or mucous membranes. In 1933 Shope and Hurst identified the first Papilloma Virus (PV) in the warty lesions of rabbits and through this investigation the suspicion of infection in warty lesions was confirmed and they concluded that the disease occurred through viral transmission.

Historically, the association between the HPV virus and cervical cancer began in 1949, when pathologist George Papanicolau introduced the most widespread test in the world for detecting the disease: the Pap smear. Through this test, it was possible to identify women with pre-malignant cellular alterations, making it possible to observe an association between sexual activity and the development of cervical cancer.

In 1950, the carcinogenic potential of human papillomavirus (HPV) was discovered in patients with epidermodysplasia verruciformis. The structure of the viral genome was only demonstrated in 1963 by Crawford & Crawford. However, in subsequent years, research into HPV was discouraged by the impossibility of a tissue culture system and the apparent benign nature of human warts.

However, it was only in the 1970s that knowledge about the etiology of the disease made considerable progress. Studies found that this association implied the presence of a sexually transmitted etiologic agent. Harold zurHausen, a German infectologist, discovered that the Human Papilloma Virus could be this agent, initially determining the virus's relationship with warts and condylomas. Only years later, the virus was linked to the development of cervical carcinoma.

In the early 1980s, there was an accelerated growth in research, HPVs 16 and 18 were identified and their relationship with cervical cancer was established. In 1987, the first epidemiological study on HPV and cervical cancer was published. From then on, several cervical molecular studies by certain types of HPV became a precursor event in the genesis of cervical neoplasia.

In 1995, the International Agency for Research on Cancer (IARC) conducted a multicenter case-control study with 2,000 cases of cervical cancer and 2,000 controls. The analysis showed a strong association between cervical cancer and the presence of any type of HPV. The *odds ratio* (OR) for all pairs adjusted for age was 60 (95%CI:49-73). The risk of an association between HPV and cervical cancer in some studies is considered to be greater than 100. No other risk factor for cervical cancer has a similar magnitude. However, HPV infection is necessary, but not sufficient, to cause cervical cancer. The vast majority of women infected with oncogenic HPV never develop cancer, indicating that additional factors must act together for the disease to develop.

Also in 1995, HPV infection was found to be the most prevalent STD (25.6%) in a heterogeneous population of adolescent women, with a large proportion of clinically unrecognized infections (24%). The most prevalent HPV types found were HPVs 16/18 (7.3%), followed by HPVs 31/33/35 (4.7%) and HPVs 6/11 (3.5%). Factors associated with the detection of HPV - DNA through multivariate analysis in studies covers number of lifetime sexual partners and warts on examination, the authors support the idea that HPV is acquired predominantly through sexual contact, and usually soon after the onset of sexual activity.

REFERENCES

ALVARENGA, G.C et al. Human papillomavirus and carcinogenesis in the cervix. **DST - Jornal Brasileiro de Doenças Sexualmente Transmissiveis**, v.12, n.1, p.2838, 2000.

CAMARA, G. N. N. L. et al. Human papillomavirus - HPV: history, morphology and biological cycle. **Universitas Ciências da Saude**, v.1, n.1, p.149-158, 2003.

CAMPOS, R. R. et al. Prevalence of human papillomavirus and its genotypes in women with and without human immunodeficiency virus. **Revista Brasileira Ginecologia e Obstetricia**, v.27, n.5, p. 248-256, 2005.

JACYNTHO, C. **HPV: the sex cancer virus? Our doubts!** Rio de Janeiro: Claudia Jacyntho, 2001. p. 28-31, 53-4.

LETO, M.G.P. et al. Human papillomavirus infection: etiopathogenesis, molecular biology and clinical manifestations. **Anais Brasileiros de Dermatologia**, v.86, n.2, p.306-317, 2011.

NAKAGAWA, J. T. T.; SCHIMER, J; BARBIERI, M. Virus HPV and cervical cancer. **Revista Brasileira de Enfermagem**, v.63, n.2, p. 307-311, 2010.

ROSA, M. R. et al. Human papillomavirus and cervical neoplasia. **Caderno Saude Publica**, v.25, n.5, p.953-964, 2009.

4

INFECTION

Lais Rocha Lima

Andressa Silva de Mesquita

HPV infection is one of the most common sexually transmitted infections (STIs) in the world. The number of women who carry the HPV DNA virus worldwide reaches 291 million, mainly among adolescents and young people with an active sex life. It is estimated that 75 to 80% of the population will be affected by at least one type of HPV in their lifetime. Around 115 million women worldwide will be infected with HPV 16 or 18 at least once in their lifetime.

HPV infection is divided into three phases: clinical, subclinical and latent. The clinical phase is detected by the visual presence of warts. The most common form is the subclinical stage, which manifests itself on the cervix in 80% of cases and is diagnosed with the help of a colposcopy. At this stage, macro papillary or micro papillary lesions are usually found, corresponding to acetowhite lesions with irregular margins and the surface can be rough, punctate or mosaic. The latent form is common in normal young individuals (20-40%), varies depending on the immune status, may regress spontaneously and is mostly asymptomatic. Diagnosis is made only by molecular biology tests. It is characterized by the presence of viral DNA in the nucleus and viral replication is related to the cell cycle of the virus without any symptoms. To date, the causes that can make this phase of the infection active are unknown. Researchers believe that physiological or pathogenic immunodepression are possible triggers.

The dynamism of HPV infection in the female genital tract comprises a wide variety of events, including latent, transient, persistent and benign warts, low-grade or high-grade squamous lesions and cervical cancer. The infection process begins with the penetration of the virus into the surface of the cervix, through lesions in the basal cells of the transformation zone of the squamous epithelium of the cervix in which the virus invades the host cell, The virus then releases its genetic material, replicating its DNA and starting its biological cycle, distributing its genetic material to two daughter cells, one of which begins the process of differentiation and cell maturation, while the other remains in the basal layer, as a reservoir of viral DNA. After inoculation, the incubation period varies from three weeks to eight months. Spontaneous regression is observed in most cases. The HPV life cycle is directly linked to the host cell's cell differentiation program. The replicative phase and protein synthesis take place in the differentiated keratinocytes of the suprabasal layers.

The time of evolution and the type of lesion correlate with the amount of viral particles detected. More recent warts have a higher viral count compared to older warts. In benign lesions, the replication of the viral genome is extra-chromosomal. In malignant lesions, the viral DNA is integrated into the chromosomes of the host cell and there is no viral replication. There is inactivation of the expression of the E2 protein, which functions as a negative regulator of the expression of the E6 and E7 oncogenes. The latter promote cell immortalization by inhibiting cell cycle regulatory proteins (p53 and pRB), which are fundamental for tumour suppression.

The infection progresses slowly (10 to 20 years), causing progressive intraepithelial changes which can evolve into intraepithelial lesions (low grade squamous intraepithelial lesion (LSIL), high grade squamous intraepithelial lesion (HSIL)). Lesions on the cervix in the non-invasive phase are easier to diagnose through pap smears and colposcopy. The acute phase is marked by the appearance of warts, mostly caused by HPVs 6 and 11. However, most HPV infections are benign and disappear spontaneously within one to five years.

HPV causes lesions on the skin or mucous membranes, which can regress as a result of action by the immune system. The virus is highly contagious, causing contamination with just one exposure. It is transmitted through direct contact with infected skin or mucous membranes. The main route is through sexual intercourse, and transmission can occur from mother to baby during pregnancy and childbirth (vertical transmission).

The clinical manifestations of HPV-related diseases vary, depending on the type of HPV and the site of inoculation, but the wart is considered the classic primary lesion of the infection. Although HPV settles in a woman's body for a long time without manifesting itself, symptoms such as bleeding, itching and pain are identified as routine symptoms of the infection. Self-examination can be crucial in recognizing active infection. Symptoms commonly found in the advanced stage include bleeding, pain during intercourse and foul-smelling discharge. Early detection of active infection is important, as late diagnosis is associated with higher rates of complications. However, failure to correctly identify the signs of active infection delays treatment and contributes to the progression of the infection. This is why women should undergo preventive examinations to screen for precursor lesions (which precede) cervical cancer, even when they are feeling well.

HPV infection is difficult to prevent because it depends on contact between diseased and healthy skin and does not depend on ejaculation. Therefore, condoms should be used throughout sexual intercourse. Avoid smoking, excessive drinking and drug use, as these activities weaken the body's defense system, making you more susceptible to HPV. In addition to routine Pap smears as a preventive test. The recent release for clinical use of vaccines against the four HPV subtypes is a breakthrough for effective HPV prevention and the prevention of anogenital cancers.

REFERENCES

ANDERSON, T. A. et al. A study of human papillomavirus on vaginally inserted sex toys, before and after cleaning, among women who have sex with men and women. **Sexually Transmitted Infections**, v. 90, n.7, p. 529-31,2014.

BUOSI, L; OLIVEIRA, L, F. C. The approach to the partner of women diagnosed with HPV. Monograph (specialization) - Secretaria de estado de saùde do Distrito Federal / **Fundaçâo de ensino e pesquisa em ciência da saude**, 2007.

BURCHELL, N. A. et al. Epidemiology and transmission dynamics of genital HPV infection. **Vaccine**, v. 24, n. 3, p.52-61, 2006.

CIRINO, F. M. S. B.; NICHIATA, L. Y. I.; BORGES, A. L. V. Knowledge, attitude and practices in the prevention of cervical cancer and hpv in adolescents. **Escola Anna Nery Revista de Enfermagem**, v.14, n.1, p. 126-34, 2010.

DOORBAR J. The papilloma viruses life cycle. **Journal of Clinical Virology**, v. 32, n.1, p. 7- 15, 2005.

FARIA, I. M. Comparative study between colpocytology and polymerase chain reaction for the diagnosis of human papilloma virus in the uterine cervix of women with human immunodeficiency virus. **Revista Brasileira de Ginecologia e Obstetricia,** v.30, n.5,p.268,2008.

HARWOOD, C. A. et al. Human papillomavirus infection and non-melanoma skin cancer in immunosuppressed and immunocompetent individuals. **Journal of Medical Virology**, v.61, n.3, p. 289-97, 2000.

KILKENNY , M.; MARKS, R. The descriptive epidemiology of warts in the community. **Australasian Journal of Dermatology**, v.37, n.2, p.80-86, 1996.

NAKAGAWA, J. T. T.; SCHIRMER, J.; BARBIERI, M. Virus HPV and cervical cancer. **Revista Brasileira de Enfermagem**, v.6, n.2, p. 307-11, 2010.

SCHIFFMAN, M. Human papillomavirus and cervical cancer. **Lancet**, v. 370, n.9590, p. 890-907, 2007.

SCHIFFMAN, M. et al. Human Papillomavirus Testing in the Prevention of Cervical Cancer. **Journal of the National Cancer Institute**, v.103, n.5, p. 368-83, 2011.

SKOCZY'NSKI, M.; GO'ZDZICKA-JÔZEFIAK, A.; KWA'SNIEWSKA, A. Risk factors of the vertical transmission of human papilloma virus in newborns from singleton pregnancy- preliminary report. **The Journal Maternal- Fetal& Neonatal Medicine**, v.27, n.3, p.239-42, 2014.

TSCHANDL, P, ROSENDAHL, C, KITTLER, H. Cutaneous human papillomavirus infection: manifestations and diagnosis. **Current Problems Dermatology**, v.45, p. 92-7, 2014.

5

EPIDEMIOLOGY OF HPV

Lais Rocha Lima

Ranyelison Silva Machado

The Human Papillomavirus (HPV) is a virus that spreads worldwide. The most common type of disease caused by it are skin warts, which have an incidence of 7 to 10% in the European population and around 1% in the American population.

In Brazil, the prevalence of high-risk HPV infection is 17.8% to 27%, being higher in women under 35 and 12% to 15% in women aged 35 to 65, while among young women aged 15 to 19 this prevalence is 43%. The incidence rate of HPV infection is around 30% to 40% in patients under the age of 20, which drops to 10% in patients over the age of 35 and the risk of infection by high-risk (oncogenic) HPV drops to 5%.

Approximately 5% to 15% of women who have not previously had contact with the HPV virus can be infected with any type of high-risk HPV, reaching a percentage of 25% where the incidence is concentrated in the 15 to 20 age group. The longest average duration of HPV infection is associated with types 16, 18, 61 and 73.

In immunosuppressed patients, these numbers tend to increase by up to 100 times, especially in kidney transplant recipients, reaching more than 90% after 15 years of the organ having been transplanted. Warts can occur in any age group, with a confirmed increase in incidence during the school period, with a peak in adolescence (from 15 to 20 years).

Incidence rates can vary greatly depending on the continent, country or region. For example, in the United States and Canada, the average incidence rate is 16.3 per 100 people per year and in Colombia it is 5 cases per 100 people per year. It is important to note that another study in Canada recorded a rate of 9.5 per person per year.

In Brazil, the incidence rate recorded until the end of the 20th century averaged 8 cases per 100 people per year. In 2008, there was a 14.3% incidence of high-risk genital HPV infection, of which 77.8% were high-grade squamous lesions and 100%

were cancer cases.

HPV 16 is one of the most common high-risk types among women and is also often the most prevalent among cervical cancer cases, reaching rates of 24.3% in women with an average age of 16 and an incidence of 24.3% in women aged 25. HPV subtype 18 is also included among the high-risk cases, with a prevalence of 7.3% in women with an average age of 16 years and close to 25 years, this rate is around 7.2%.

The World Health Organization (WHO) estimates that 630 million men and women are infected with this virus worldwide. In Brazil, it is estimated that 700,000 new cases are emerging, which could be considered an epidemic.

In Brazil, the National Cancer Institute (INCA) is the body that helps the Ministry of Health to coordinate integrated actions for the prevention and control of cancer in the country, and it also publishes epidemiological results and future estimates. In 2018, according to INCA, the incidence rate of cervical cancer in Brazil was 17.11 cases per 100,000 women, and the mortality rate was 4.7 deaths per 100,000 women.

In the United States, this rate is 15/100,000 for the white population alone and 34/100,000 for the black population. The WHO estimates that there are 500,000 new cases of cervical cancer every year and that half of the women who are affected could die. It is the cause of 11% of cancers in women worldwide.

It is known that every 2 minutes a woman dies of cervical cancer in the world. Thus, if trends continue, the outlook is for 1 million new cases every year by 2050.

The HPV subtypes that present a high oncogenic risk are types 16, 18, 31, 35, 45, 51, 52, 58 and 59, which are more prevalent in Africa and Latin America. HPV 16 is the most common subtype in the world. HPV 18 is the most common in Indonesia and Algeria and in West Africa HPV 45 is the most prevalent. Types 33, 39 and 59 can be found more easily in Central and South America.

It is therefore clear that the incidence of HPV is on the rise and that it occurs in almost the same proportion worldwide, affecting men, women, children and adults. It is known that the peak of this incidence occurs between the ages of 20 and 40, with one of the main reasons being the beginning of adulthood, as well as factors such as shyness, lack of knowledge or even fear. In conclusion, due to the high incidence rates of HPV infection, it has become an important public health problem and requires a great deal of attention.

REFERENCES

CARDOSO, E. M. M. **Historical, physiopathological and preventive aspects of Human Papilloma Virus - HPV infection**. 2012. Course Conclusion Paper (Specialization) - Nescon, Federal University of Minas Gerais, Minas Gerais.

CARVALHO, J. J. M; OYAKAWA, N. **I Congresso Brasileiro de HPV - Papilomavirus Humano.** 1ª edition. Sâo Paulo: BG Cultural, 2000.

FERLAY, J. et al. Globocan 2002 cancer incidence: Mortality and prevalence worldwide. **IARC Cancer Base**, v. 5, p. 123-129, 2004.

FRANCO, E. L. et al. Epidemiology of acquisition and clearance of cervical human papillomavirus infection in women from a high-risk area for cervical cancer. **Journal of Infectious Diseases**, v. 182, p. 1415-1423, 1999.

HENGGE, U. R. Papilloma virus diseases. **Hautarzt**, v. 55, p. 841-851, 2004.

HO, G. Y. et al. Natural history of cervicovaginal papillomavirus infection in young women. **New England Journal of Medicine,** v. 338, n. 7, p. 423-428, 1998.

HOSSNE, R. S. Prevalence of asymptomatic perianal papilloma virus (HPV) in patients with genital HPV treated at the Hospital das Clinicas da Faculdade de Medicina de Botucatu. **Revista Brasileira de Coloproctologia**, v. 28, n. 2, p. 223226, 2008.

IARC. **International Agency for Research on Cancer**. Handbooks of Cancer Prevention: Cervix Cancer Screening. Lyon: IARC, 2005.

INCA, José Alencar Gomes da Silva Cancer Institute. **2016 estimate, Cancer incidence in Brazil**. Available at: http://www.inca.gov.br/bvscontrolecancer/publicacoes/edicao/Estimativa_2016.pdf. Accessed on: December 21, 2018.

KILKENNY, M.; MARKS, R. The descriptive epidemiology of warts in the community. **Australasian Journal of Dermatology**, v. 37, p. 80-86, 1996.

LINDELOF, B. et al. Incidence of skin cancer in 5356 patients following organ transplantation. **British Journal of Dermatology**, v. 143, p. 614-618, 2000.

RAMA, C. H. et al. HPV prevalence in women screened for cervical cancer. **Revista Saude Publica**, v. 42, n. 1, p. 123-130, 2008.

RIVERA, Z. et al. Epidemiology of the human papilloma virus (HPV). **Revista**

Chilena de Obstetricia e Ginecologia, v. 67, n. 6, p. 501-506, 2002.

SELLORS, J. W. et al. Incidence, clearance and predictors of human papillomavirus infection in women. **Canadian Medical Association Journal**, v. 168, n. 4, p. 168174,2003

6

HPV VACCINE

Ivisson Lucas Campos da Silva

Lais Rocha Lima

Persistent infection of cervical epithelial cells with high-risk carcinogenic types of HPV causes 99% of the estimated 530,000 global cases of cervical cancer that occur each year, even more so in underdeveloped countries where screening and treatment programs are ineffective or often non-existent. Among the different types of HPVs, two (subtypes 16 and 18) account for 70% of the causes of cancer worldwide (20% and 50% of cervical cancers, respectively) and five high-risk HPV subtypes are responsible for approximately 90% of the global burden of cervical cancer. It is therefore not surprising that the first HPV vaccines were targeted at these genotypes.

According to the World Health Organization (WHO), it is recommended that all countries include the HPV vaccine in the immunization schedule, establishing the following program: two doses for girls aged 9 to 14, with a minimum interval of 6 months and 3 doses for girls aged 15 and over. It is worth noting that vaccination is not recommended for pregnant women, despite the literature indicating that there are no risks or adverse effects in pregnancy. In addition, young immunocompromised individuals should be vaccinated with 3 doses.

If the vaccination schedule is interrupted, it should not be restarted. If there is an interruption after the first dose, the second dose should be administered as soon as possible, and the interval between the second and third doses may be reduced to three months. If only the third dose is overdue, it should be administered as soon as possible. It's worth noting that the Ministry of Health has extended immunization to boys aged between 11 and 15. Since January 2019, the vaccine in question has been available on the Unified Health System (SUS) for boys aged 12 to 13. Until then, it was only given to girls under the age of 15.

According to data from the National Immunization Program Information System (SI-PNI), in 2014, 5,354,224 girls aged 11-13 received their first dose of the vaccine: an estimated coverage of 108.0%. However, only 60.1% returned to the vaccination center after 6 months for the second dose. Vaccination is characterized as primary prevention, but it does not replace Pap smears or condom use, as it does not prevent 30% of cervical cancer cases caused by other oncogenic viral subtypes. The expectation is that in the next 10 to 20 years after the vaccine is implemented, there will be a reduction in the incidence rates of precursor lesions of cervical cancer.

In 2006, the National Health Surveillance Agency (ANVISA) approved two prophylactic vaccines against HPV. However, both were only available in private healthcare institutions. After careful evaluation by the Brazilian Ministry of Health, in 2014 the quadrivalent HPV vaccine (Gardasil) was included in the national immunization program for girls between 11 and 13 years of age.

Many of the developing countries with the highest incidence rates of cervical cancer have not yet introduced HPV vaccination into the immunization schedule. Given this current scenario, the Centers for Disease Control and Prevention (CDC) is committed to supporting vaccine introduction in these locations, including laboratory evaluation of HPV vaccines, training of field epidemiologists and advancement of cervical cancer registries, as these efforts contribute to global health security.

The current vaccines against HPV (Gardasil and Cervarix) aim to combat the spread of the virus and control virus-induced lesions. Both are made up of virus-like particles (VLPs) derived from the virus's large capsid protein (L1), which are morphologically similar to the virus without, however, containing viral DNA. The gene encoding the L1 protein of each type is expressed in the yeast *Saccharomyces cerevisiae*. Both vaccines have a high immunogenic capacity and produce long-lasting antibody responses.

These prophylactic vaccines stimulate a humoral response based on contact with VLPs. The expression of capsid proteins (L1 and L2) generates VLPs, which are considered the main sources of antigens used in clinical tests for the development of prophylactic vaccines. In this way, the antibodies produced by the vaccine are released into the genital mucosa, which prevents the early formation of an infection.

In addition to subtypes 16 and 18, the quadrivalent vaccine also prevents infections with subtypes 6 and 11, and is effective against half of all infections with subtype 31. Although the vaccines provide strong protection against oncogenic HPV types, they offer little cross-protection against other high-risk HPV types.

It is worth noting that Brazil is one of the countries with wide vaccination coverage, given its ability to effectively vaccinate against all types of HPV. One way of achieving broad vaccination coverage is to produce a multivalent vaccine, containing the eight most common HPV virus subtypes, so that it can achieve greater than 90% protection against cervical cancer. However, its limitation is based on the high cost of the vaccine, since the current ones against the HPV virus are already very expensive. As a result, the vaccine may not be affordable in low- and middle-income countries. Another limitation to be emphasized is the transport and storage of current HPV vaccines, since in underdeveloped or developing countries, refrigerated facilities are often inadequate.

REFERENCES

De MARTEL, C. et al. Worldwide burden of cancer attributable to HPV by site, country and HPV type. **International Journal of Cancer**, v. 141, n. 4, p. 664-670, 2017.

World Health Organization (WHO). Human papillomavirus vaccines: WHO position paper, May 2017. **The Wkly Epidemiological Record**, v. 92, n. 19, p. 241-68, 2017.

SERRANO, B. et al. Human papillomavirus genotype attribution for HPVs 6, 11, 16, 18, 31, 33, 45, 52 and 58 in female genital lesions. **European Journal of Cancer**, v. 51, n. 13, p. 1732-41, 2015.

Skeate, J. G. et al. Current therapeutic vaccination and immunotherapy strategies for HPV-related diseases. **Human Vaccines & Immuno therapeutics**, v. 12, n. 6, p. 1418-29, 2016.

MARKOWITZ, L. E. et al. Quadrivalent human papillomavirus vaccine: recommendations of the Advisory Committee on Immunization Practices (ACIP). **MMWR Recommendations and Reports**, v. 56, n. RR-2, p. 1-24, 2007.

Ministry of Health (BR). Information System of the National Immunization Program. HPV vaccination strategy [Internet]. Brasilia: Ministério da Saùde; 2014 [cited 2018 Dec 26] Available from:
http : //pni.datasus .gov.br/consulta_hpv_ 14_C01 .php.

KURY, C. M. et al. Implementation of the quadrivalent vaccine against HPV in the Municipality of Campos dos Goytacazes, Brazil - A combinationofstrategiestoincreaseimmunizationcoverageandearlyreductionof genital warts. **Trials in Vaccinology**, n. 2, p. 1924, 2013.

World Health Organization (WHO). Immunization vaccines and biological database, April 2017. Geneva: The Organization; 2017.

Centers for Disease Control and Prevention. CDC' s strategic framework for global immunization, 2016-2020, 2016. Available at:
<https: //www.cdc. gov/globalhealth/immunization/docs/global-immunization-framework-508.pdf> Accessed 24 July 2018.

KIM, K. S. et al. Current status of human papilloma virus vaccines. **Clinical and Experimental Vaccine Research**, v.3, n.2, p. 168-75, 2014.

TYLER, M; TUMBAN, E; CHACKERIAN, B. Second-generation prophylactic HPV vaccines: successes and challenges. **Expert Review Vaccines**, v. 13, n.2, p. 247-55,

2 014.

SCHILLER, J. T.; CASTELLSAGUÉ, X.; GARLAND, S. M. A review of clinical trials of human papilloma virus prophylactic vaccines. **Vaccine**, v. 30, n. 5, p.123-38, 2012.

GUPTA G.; GLUECK, R; PATEL, P. R. HPV vaccines: Global perspectives. **Human Vaccines & Immuno therapeutics**, v. 13, n. 6, p. 1-4, 2017.

TUMBAN, E. et al. Preclinical refinements of a broadly protective VLP-based HPV vaccine targeting the minor capsid protein, L2. **Vaccine**, v. 33, n. 29, p. 3346-3353, 2 015.

CERVANTES, J. L.; DOAN, A. H. Discrepancies in the evaluation of the safety of the human papilloma virus vaccine. **Memorias do Instituto Oswaldo Cruz**, v. 113, n. 8, e180063, 2018.

RODEN, R; WU, T. C. How will HPV vaccines affect cervical cancer? **Nature Reviews Cancer**, v. 6, n. 10, p. 753- 763, 2006.

7

DIAGNOSIS

Lais Rocha Lima

Talita Pereira Lima da Silva

Cervical-vaginal cytology was introduced by George Papanicolau and Aurel Babes in 1928. In 1943, the method was recognized as being excellent for the prevention and early diagnosis of cervical cancer. The introduction of this diagnostic test reduced mortality rates from cervical cancer by around 50% to 70%. Its effectiveness is nationally recognized.

This test is carried out by collecting and analyzing cellular samples from the ectocervix and endocervix, the inner and outer parts of the cervix, identifying the presence of possible cellular alterations and precancerous lesions, providing an initial diagnosis of the disease, even before symptoms appear. This procedure is a simple, reliable and low-cost method that can be carried out by any health professional as long as they are qualified. It is a screening method, not a definitive diagnosis, and is carried out routinely in the primary health care network.

The cytopathology test is carried out with the woman in the gynecological position. The professional introduces the speculum into the vaginal canal to make it easier to see the cervix, then introduces the Ayres spatula to collect the material from the ectocervix. The material collected needs to be placed in only half of the space on the slide, and deposited transversely. Subsequently, the cervical brush is introduced into the uterine canal to collect material from the endocervix, placing it longitudinally on the part of the slide that is still free of material, using a rotating motion, followed by fixing the cytological material on the slide and cell staining.

The cytological examination of the uterine cervix is of great importance for screening pre-cancerous lesions on the cervix. It is a secondary prevention strategy, and its performance is essential for the early diagnosis of the neoplasm. The identification of the disease at an early stage, that is, before the lesions become invasive, and the prognosis of cure can reach 100%. It is recommended for women aged 25 to 64 every three years, after two consecutive negative cytology results.

Women who have already started sexual activity are advised to have two tests at one-year intervals with negative results, and the next tests should be carried out every three years. This test should be stopped when the patient reaches the age of 64 with no previous history of pre-neoplasic lesions and has had two consecutive negative tests in the last five years.

There are still some issues of resistance or non-performance on the part of women, including age, marital status, schooling and income, cultural issues such as fear of pain, shame, lack of knowledge of the procedure, the place where it is carried out and discouragement on the part of the partner.

The cytopathology test is carried out in two ways: conventional and in liquid form. Through this test we can detect morphological changes in cells related to the cytopathic effect of HPV infection, such as: the presence of cells with irregular cavities around the nucleus (koilocytes), characterizing the cytopathic effect caused by HPV (koilocytosis), cytomegaly, multinucleation, hyperchromasia, atypical parakeratosis, irregular contour of the nuclear membrane and perinuclear halo.

The conventional method has disadvantages in some of the test procedures, such as the subjectivity of the reading of the material collected, errors at the time of collection and also in the fixation of the material. A large number of unsatisfactory tests with false-negative results are observed.

The liquid method was developed to reduce the shortcomings of conventional cytology. It produces a slide with a cleaner background, without overlapping cells or obscuring other elements, retaining only the epithelial cells, facilitating diagnosis.

Its advantages include better preservation of the cells, improving the quality of the material to be analyzed, reducing analysis time by 30%, greater productivity, a reduction in the number of false-negative results and unsatisfactory smears, as well as the preservation of 100% of the material collected in the fixative liquid for possible histochemical or molecular biology tests. The disadvantages of this method are the high cost of the equipment, its maintenance and the training of professionals to carry out the reading.

Another test carried out in association with cytology is oncotic colpocytology, which is characterized as the most effective method for screening for cervical cancer by means of a careful visual analysis of the cervix and vagina to observe precancerous lesions. Its purpose is to confirm the diagnosis of pre-neoplastic lesions and for secondary prevention. It takes place by means of a smear or scraping of exfoliated cells from the cervical and vaginal epithelium, and if any alterations are found, a biopsy is recommended.

The histological examination is carried out on material taken from the biopsy, which consists of removing one or more fragments of the altered area of the cervix. Colposcopy makes it possible to evaluate and exclude micro-invasive or glandular diseases, by means of an anatomopathological analysis of the sample taken from the lesion, confirming and grading the stage of the lesion.

Detection of the HPV virus and its genetic material (DNA) is carried out using hybridization tests, the dot blot and reverse blot, which have good accuracy and sensitivity, but are more demanding techniques. Southern blot has good sensitivity and specificity and estimates the amount of DNA in the lesion, while in situ hybridization allows the topographic location of viral DNA in cells and tissues using radiolabelled probes. These tests identify the virus even in asymptomatic patients and help monitor and treat precursor lesions of cervical cancer.

The PCR technique consists of amplifying the target DNA sequence in millions of times to determine the HPV genotype present in clinical samples from the genital mucosa, verifying whether the HPVs are of high or low risk for the development of cervical neoplasms, as well as helping to choose the most appropriate therapeutic approach for patients.

Other techniques used to identify HPV are genotyping techniques, which are used to assess the prognosis of epithelial lesions on the cervix, identify HPV types, high-risk groups and factors associated with regression, progression and persistence of cervical HPV infection.

The PapilloCheck, Greinerbio-one®, Monroe, NC brands perform simultaneous genotyping of 24 types of HPV, high-risk (HPVs 16, 18, 31, 33, 35, 39, 45, 51, 52, 53, 66, 56, 58, 59, 68, 70, 73 and 82) and low-risk (HPVs 6, 11, 40, 42,

43, 44 and 55). Another methodology is the molecular hybrid capture II (CH II) test for HPV, which is a reference in complementing the diagnosis of HPV infections and is recommended as an adjunct to the Pap smear. It detects the DNA of 18 viral types with a sensitivity of 91.7% and specificity of 95.4%.

Combining cytology with molecular biology can increase the sensitivity and negative predictive value to around 100%, suggesting that women with negative results from both tests can be re-screened at longer intervals. However, gynecologists recommend visits every six months, with annual cytology and colposcopy or hybrid capture. This approach is only considered when the cytology shows a low-grade intraepithelial lesion, the initial colposcopy is satisfactory and the biopsy confirms CIN I.

In order to standardize the diagnosis of cervical lesions, a meeting of specialists was held in Maryland, USA, in 1982, when the Bethesda System was created. This established cytological classification standards in order to reduce diagnostic contradictions between benign and atypical cellular alterations and the cytological terms of low-grade intraepithelial lesion, comprising alterations suggestive of HPV infection and grade I intraepithelial neoplasia (CIN I), high-grade intraepithelial lesions, such as cytological expressions of CIN II and III, and atypical squamous cells of undetermined significance (ASCUS), defined by the presence of cytological findings insufficient for the diagnosis of intraepithelial lesions.

In 2001, a meeting of experts was held in Bethesda at which the ASCUS category was revised because it presented limitations in terms of cytological changes that were reparative or neoplasic, which led to the reclassification into "ASCUS" - "atypical squamous cells of undetermined significance" and "ASC-H" - "atypical squamous cells that cannot be excluded from high-grade intraepithelial lesions"

REFERENCES

DAVIM, R. M. B. et al. Knowledge of women from a Basic Health Unit in the city of Natal/RN about the Pap smear. **Revista Escola de Enfermagem USP**, Sâo Paulo, v.39, n.3, p.296-30, 2005.

DERCHAIN, S. F. M; LONGATTO, A.F; SYRJANEN, K. J. Cervical intraepithelial neoplasia: diagnosis and treatment. **Revista Brasileira de Ginecologia e Obstetricia**, v.27, n.7, p.425-33, 2005.

FERREIRA, M. L. S. M. Motives that influence the non-realization of the Pap smear according to the perception of women. **Escola Anna Nery**, v.13, n. 2, p. 37884, 2009.

FREITAS, T. P. et al. Molecular detection of HPV 16 and 18 in cervical samples of patients from Belo Horizonte, Minas Gerais, Brazil. **Revista do Instituto de Medicina Tropical**, v.49, n.5, p. 297-301, 2007.

GRAVITT, P. E. et al. A comparison between real-time polymerase chain reaction and hybrid capture 2 for human Papillomavirus DNA quantification. **Cancer Epidemiology Biomarkers & Prevention**, v.12, n.6, p.477-84, 2003.

KARNON, J. et al. Liquid-based cytology in cervical screening: an updated rapid and systematic review and economic analysis. **Health Technology Assessment**, v.8, n.20, p. 1-78, 2004.

LETO, M. G. P. et al. Human papillomavirus infection: etiopathogenesis, molecular biology and clinical manifestations. **Anais Brasileiros de Dermatologia**, v.86, n.2, p.306-17,2011.

MITTELDORF, C. A. T. S. Cervical cancer screening: from Pap smear to future strategies. **Brazilian Journal of Pathology and Laboratory Medicine**, v. 52, n.4, p.238-45, 2016.

MOURA, E. R. F. et al. Clinical, therapeutic and sexual panorama of women with Human Papilloma Virus and/or Cervical Intraepithelial Neoplasia. **Revista de Enfermagem Referência**, v.4, n.3, p.113-120, 2014.

NONNENMACHERA, B. et al. Identification of human papillomavirus by molecular biology in asymptomatic women. **Revista de Saude Publica**, v.36, n.1, p. 95100, 2002.

PIMENTEL, A. V. et al. The perception of vulnerability among women diagnosed with advanced cervical cancer. **Texto Contexto Enfermagem**, V. 20, n. 2, p. 255-62,

2011.

ROCHA, J. M.; SANTOS, V. L. O.; CUNHA, K. J. B. Cervical Cancer: Challenges for Early Diagnosis. **Revista Saùde em Foco**, v.1, n2, p.1-11, 2014.

STABILE, S. A. B. et al. Comparative study of the results obtained by conventional cervical-vaginal oncology cytology and liquid-based cytology. **Einstein**, v.10, n.4, p.466-72, 2012.

SILVA, E. R. et al. Molecular diagnosis of HPV by hybrid capture and polymerase chain reaction. **Femina**, v.43, n.4, p.181-184, 2015.

SILVA, D. S. M. et al. Cervical Cancer Screening in the State of Maranhâo, Brazil. **Ciência e Saùde Coletiva**, v. 19, n. 4, p. 1163-1170, 2014.

SOUSA, A. N. L. et al. Cytopathic effects of human papillomavirus infection and the severity of cervical intraepithelial neoplasia: A frequency study. **Diagnostic Cytopathology**, v.40, n.10, p.871-5, 2011.

THOMISON, J.; THOMAS, L. K; SHROYER, K.R. Human papillomavirus: molecular and cytologic/histologic aspects related to cervical intraepithelial neoplasia and carcinoma. **Human Pathology**, v, 39, n.2, p.154-66, 2008.

TUON, F. F. B. et al. Evaluation of the sensitivity and specificity of cytopathologic and colposcopic examinations in relation to histologic examination in the identification of cervical intraepithelial lesions. **Revista da Associaçâo Medica Brasileira**, v.48, n.2, p. 140-4 2002.

TULIO, S. et al. Relationship between the viral load of oncogenic HPV determined by the hybrid capture method and the cytological diagnosis of high-grade lesions. **Brazilian Journal of Pathology and Laboratory Medicine**, v.43, n.1, p. 31-35, 2007.

VILLA, L. L. et al. Molecular variants of human papillomavirus types 16 and 18 preferentially associated with cervical neoplasia. **Journal of General Virology**, v.81, n.12, p.2959-68, 2000.

8

TREATMENT

Lais Rocha Lima

Thalia Pires do Nascimento

Cervical intraepithelial neoplasia can progress to more serious lesions or invasive carcinoma. This progression depends on the degree or severity of the lesion. The greater the degree of abnormality of the histological examination result, the greater the rate of progression to a more severe lesion and the faster. For all women diagnosed with CIN 1, 2 or 3, regular follow-up is necessary. CIN 1 can only be managed by observational follow-up. CIN 2 is likely to regress without treatment, as this has occurred in a large number of women. CIN 3 cases require treatment to completely destroy the abnormal epithelium, preferably excision of the cervix or conization. In adult women diagnosed with HSIL who cannot identify CIN 2 or CIN 3 histologically, excisional diagnosis or observation by colposcopy and cytology at intervals of six months to one year is recommended.

Treatment for early-stage disease (1 or 2a) is usually surgical, unless there are contraindications. Surgeries range from a cone biopsy for early stage 1a to a radical hysterectomy (total removal of the uterus). The
Fertility-sparing surgeries are increasingly being used in less advanced stages, such as laparoscopy, trachelectomy or radical trachelectomy for selected cases and have excellent results, but are not available in most developing countries.

For histologically confirmed cases of HSIL, the Australian Consensus recommends ablative treatment, which can be carried out using a carbon dioxide laser. The treatment must be carried out according to the following criteria: a targeted biopsy that confirms the diagnosis, no evidence of invasive cancer on cytology, colposcopy or biopsy, and no glandular lesion on cytology or biopsy. European guidelines recommend that women treated for HSIL require cytological follow-up at 6, 12 and 24 months, followed by annual cytology for a period of 5 years. Colposcopy should be performed together with cytology at the sixth month follow-up visit.

In cases of cervical cancer (CC), colposcopy determines the best course of action, which can range from simply repeating the oncologic colposcopy exam in six months, to surgical treatment or RT, which uses ionizing radiation to fight neoplasms, preventing the multiplication of malignant cells by mitosis and/or determining cell death. Chemotherapy is not the treatment of choice for CC, but current treatment protocols have recommended its concomitant use with radiotherapy, increasing the response to therapy. This treatment has increased the overall survival rate of patients (65%), ranging from 15% to 80%, depending on the extent of the disease. Radiotherapy consists of radiation from an external pelvic beam with high-energy photons and intracavitary brachytherapy. Although the increased dose of radiation increases the control of the pathology, the dose should be administered with caution due to the possibility of late complications. Even if the treatment is effective, many cells seek out resistance mechanisms, such as hypoxia, which makes it necessary to combine it with chemotherapy. The standard chemotherapy drug of choice is cisplastin, which, despite its excellent antineoplastic activity, generally induces nephrotoxicity and gastrointestinal toxicity. Neoadjuvant chemotherapy can be used before radical surgery, as it can help reduce the tumor.

A complementary therapy, still experimental, called regional hyperthermia, has shown promise in the treatment of cervical cancer. This therapy should be carried out in conjunction with chemotherapy and radiotherapy. It is based on raising the temperature of the tumor to 40-43°C. In studies, hyperthermic radiochemotherapy has been shown to improve the prognosis of patients with CC.

REFERENCES

BRAZIL. José Alencar Gomes da Silva National Cancer Institute. Coordination of Prevention and Surveillance. Division of Early Detection and Support for Network Organization. Brazilian guidelines for cervical cancer screening. - 2. ed. rev. atual. - Rio de Janeiro: INCA, 2016.

COLOMBO, N. et al. Cervical cancer: ESMO Clinical Practice Guidelines for diagnosis, treatment and follow-up. **Annals of oncology**, v. 23, n.7, p. 27-32, 2012

DENNY, L. Cervical cancer: prevention and treatment. **Discovery medicine**, v. 14, n. 75, p. 125-131, 2012.

OLIVEIRA, P.S. et al. Management of high-grade intraepithelial lesions in adult women. **Revista do Colégio Brasileiro de Cirurgiôes**, v. 38, n. 4, p. 274-279, 2011.

9

CERVICAL CANCER

Aniclécio Mendes Lima

Lais Rocha Lima

Mariana Dantas Coutinho

Cervical cancer (CC) is a serious public health problem in developing countries. It is one of the biggest indicators of morbidity and mortality among women from lower social classes, since these women live in regions where the health services network is precarious, especially when it comes to detecting and treating the pathology and its precursor lesions.

Currently, this neoplasm is feared by women because the uterus is significant in women's lives, as it represents sexuality, femininity and the ability to reproduce. In this context, the diagnosis of CC causes biological, psychological, social and spiritual changes in the lives of women and their families.

Cervical cancer is asymptomatic or has few symptoms in its early stages. It develops in the cervix, radiating to the vagina, cervical and parametrial tissues, and can affect the bladder, ureters and rectum. The distant spread of this disease occurs via the lymphatic route, affecting pelvic and para-aortic lymph nodes.

The clinical presentation depends mainly on the location and extent of the disease. Symptoms usually appear late, when the cancer has invaded other tissues or organs, such as: minor bleeding outside the menstrual period, longer and more voluminous periods than usual, bleeding after sexual intercourse, douching or vaginal examination, pain during intercourse, bleeding after the menopause and increased vaginal discharge.

Cervical cancer is a slow-developing disease that usually affects women over the age of 25. It is characterized by the disordered replication of the organ's lining epithelium, involving the underlying tissue (stroma) and may metastasize to nearby or distant organs and structures. Carcinoma of the cervix is subdivided into two categories according to the origin of the epithelium involved: squamous cell carcinoma, which is more common and accounts for around 80% of cases, mainly affecting the squamous epithelium, and adenocarcinoma, which is rarer and affects the glandular epithelium, accounting for around 10% of cases.

Cervical cancer neoplasms originate in the epithelium lining the ectocervix or in the epithelial cells lining the glands of the endocervix. The development of cervical cancer is very slow and goes through many stages, from pre-clinical to detectable and curable. According to the National Cancer Institute (INCA) there are several factors in the development of cervical cancer, and the HPV virus (human papillomavirus) with its oncogenic subtypes is the main risk factor for the development of this neoplasm. Other factors associated with the onset of cervical cancer include early onset of sexual activity, a high number of sexual partners throughout life, immunosuppressed patients, use of immunosuppressive drugs also present an increased risk of this neoplasm, poor or lack of intimate hygiene, prolonged use of contraceptives, nulliparity, multiparity. In addition, smoking or exposure to the tobacco environment is another important factor, as the specific carcinogenic agents in tobacco, in contact with mucus and cervical epithelium, can cause DNA damage to the cells of the cervix, leading to the neoplasm process.

Cervical cancer is the fourth most common type of cancer among women, with around 530,000 new cases a year worldwide, with the exception of non-melanoma skin cancer, and the age group most affected by CC is between 30 and 49 years old. This neoplasm is the fourth most frequent cause of cancer death in women, accounting for 265,000 deaths a year. In 2016, there were 5,847 deaths from this neoplasm, giving an adjusted mortality rate for the world population of 4.70 deaths per 100,000 women.

According to the World Health Organization, as of 2020, it is estimated that 15 million new cases of uterine cancer will be diagnosed each year worldwide, with around 70% of this neoplasm occurring in countries where only 5% have the resources to control the disease. With regard to HPV infection, which is the main factor in CC, around 291 million women in the world will have it at some point in their lives, corresponding to a prevalence of 10.4%. However, more than 90% of these new infections regress spontaneously within six to eighteen months.

Cervical cancer control has been defined as a priority on the country's health agenda and is part of the Strategic Action Plan to Combat Chronic Non-Communicable Diseases (CNCD) due to its high incidence, morbidity and mortality. The Ministry of Health, in its publication "Guidelines for Cervical Cancer Screening 2016", suggests that asymptomatic women between the ages of 25 and 64 should have a cytopathological examination every three years, after two consecutive normal annual examinations. In the case of women with low-grade lesions, it recommends repeating the test in six months.

REFERENCES

ANDRADE, J. M. et al. Screening, diagnosis and treatment of cervical carcinoma. **Projeto Diretrizes [online]**, 2001.

BRASIL. **Prevençâo do câncer do colo utero**: manual técnico: profissionais de saù. Brasilia, DF, 2002. [access in August 01, 2019]. Available at: <http://bvsms.saude.gov.br/bvs/publicacoes/inca/manual_profissionaisdesaude.pdf>.

BRAZIL. National Cancer Institute - INCA. **National Cervical Cancer Control Program. Brazil**, 2011c. [access on August 02, 2019]. Available at: <http://www 1. inca.gov.br/inca/Arquivos/PROGRAMA_UTERO_internet.PDF>.

BRAZIL. Ministry of Health. Health Care Secretariat. National Cancer Institute. **Cervical cancer: technical and managerial information and actions taken**. Rio de Janeiro, 2002.

DE ATENÇÂO BÂSICA, Cadernos. Control of cervical and breast cancers. **Brasilia: Ministry of Health**, 2013.

DE ATENÇÂO BÂSICA, Cadernos. Control of cervical and breast cancers. **Brasilia: Ministry of Health**, 2006.
DIZ, M. P. E; DE MEDEIROS, R. B. Cancer of the uterine cervix - risk factors, prevention, diagnosis and treatment. **Revista de Medicina**, v. 88, n. 1, p. 7-15, 2009.

José Alencar Gomes da Silva National Cancer Institute. **Brazilian guidelines for cervical cancer screening: 2016 update**. Rio de Janeiro: INCA; 2016 [access on August 01, 2019]. Available at: http://www2.inca.gov.br/wps/wcm/connect/agencianoticias/site/home/noticias/2016/d iretrizes_para_rastreamento_cancer_colo_utero_consulta_publica.

José Alencar Gomes da Silva National Cancer Institute. **Estimate 2018: cancer incidence in Brazil**. Rio de Janeiro: INCA, 2017.

SALES, L. K. O. **Study of survival and prognostic factors in women with cervical cancer in Rio Grande do Norte, Brazil**. 2015. Master's thesis.

TSUCHIYA, C. T. et al. Cervical cancer in Brazil: a retrospective on public policies aimed at women's health. **JBES: Brazilian Journal of Health Economics**, v. 9, n. 1, 2017.

VERAS, J. M. M. F.; NERY, I. S. O significado do diagnostico de câncer do colo uterino para a mulher. **Revista Interdisciplinar NOVAFAPI**, v. 4, n. 4, p. 13-18, 2011.

10

CERVICAL CANCER IN THE WORLD AND IN BRAZIL

Lais Rocha Lima

Larruama Soares Figueiredo de Araujo

Cancer is the name given to a group of more than one hundred types of disease, the main characteristic of which is the growth of abnormal cells with invasive potential that compromise adjacent tissues and organs. Its etiology is multifactorial and can be external or internal to the body. Predisposing factors can act together or in sequence to initiate or promote carcinogenesis. When the tumor is detected early, there is a better chance of treating the disease and, consequently, curing it.

The impact of cancer on the world stage makes it a public health problem to be tackled, mainly due to the gradual increase in the incidence and mortality of patients with the disease, which is proportional to demographic growth, the ageing of the population, socio-economic development and the difficulty in guaranteeing the population full and equal access to diagnosis and treatment, since access to and use of services depends on the supply and behavior of people in the face of the disease and the services.

According to the José Alencar Gomes da Silva National Cancer Institute (INCA) there is a growing increase in estimates for new cases of cancer. In Brazil, 600,000 new cases are expected in the 2018-2019 biennium and, worldwide, by 2025, the estimate is 25 million new cases of cancer.

Cervical cancer, with almost 550,000 new cases a year worldwide, has high incidence and mortality rates. Despite being preventable, it ranks fourth among the most common types of cancer among women, and is responsible for approximately 265,000 deaths a year.

Its incidence increases in developing countries, especially low-income countries, where it ranks at the top of all female cancers, while in developed countries it ranks only sixth. The lowest rates are found in the United States, Canada, Japan, Australia and European countries. Around 85% of cervical cancer cases, according to Globocan, occur in less developed countries such as those in Latin America, the

Caribbean, Africa and South and Southeast Asia and mortality varies by up to 18 times between different regions of the world, with rates ranging from less than 2 per 100,000 women in West Asia to 27.6 in East Africa.

In Brazil, it is estimated that 15,590 women fall ill each year, with a crude incidence rate of 15.33/100,000. It is the fourth leading cause of death among women due to cancer and the second most diagnosed tumor in women, affecting them in the 20-29 age group, with a higher risk in the 45-49 age group due to the prolonged period of sexual transmission of HPV. Illness and death from cervical cancer ranks first among women in the North, in the Northeast and Midwest, second in the North and third and fourth in the Southeast and South.

In the less developed regions of Brazil, where social inequalities are marked, preventable and curable cancers are the most common. In the North, cervical cancer incidence rates are much higher than the world average, on a par with Central America, with 23.97 cases per 100,000 women. In the Southeast and South, cervical cancer has rates of 11.3/100,000 and 15.17/100,000 respectively, but breast, colon and rectum, and lung cancers predominate, which brings them closer to the profile of developed countries. In the Center-West region, the rates are 20.72 cases per 100,000 women. In the Northeast, although breast cancer has a higher incidence of 19.49/100,000, cervical cancer rates exceed the world average, bringing it closer to less developed regions.

In the Brazilian states of Amazonas, Amapa and Maranhão, the incidence of cervical cancer is similar to that of less developed countries. Cervical cancer in Amazonas is similar to the incidence in East Africa, considered one of the least developed places in the world. Amapa, Maranhão and Tocantins also have rates similar to those in African regions, especially southern and central Africa. All the states in the North, Northeast and Center-West regions (with the exception of the Federal District) have an overall incidence similar to the least developed countries. Only the states of the Southeast have rates comparable to those of the more developed countries.

In Brazil, mortality from this neoplasm reached 5,727 deaths in 2015. Data from the National Cancer Institute (INCA) for 2016 estimated 16,340 new cases (a crude incidence of approximately 16 cases per 100,000 women) and 5,340 deaths associated with CC in Brazil. There has been a reduction in mortality from cervical cancer in the country, except in some municipalities in the North and Northeast regions.

Although the incidence of cervical cancer has been falling around the world and is a preventable cause of death among women, its incidence is still high in regions with great social inequality. It is estimated that 85% of cases occur in developing countries, and women with lower incomes, low levels of education and more difficult access to health services are the most likely to die from this neoplasm. However, screening programs, access to early diagnosis and timely treatment should be implemented.

REFERENCES

BEZERRA, J.S.S. et al. Profile of women with cervical lesions caused by HPV in terms of risk factors for cervical cancer. **DST - Jornal Brasileiro de Doenças Sexualmente Transmissiveis**, v.17, n. 2, p. 143-148, 2005.

BRAZIL. Ministry of Health. Health Care Secretariat. National Cancer Institute. **Cervical cancer: technical and managerial information and actions taken.** Rio de Janeiro, 2002.

BRAZIL. Ministry of Health. José Alencar Gomes da Silva National Cancer Institute (INCA). **ABC of Cancer: Basic Approaches to Cancer Control**. Rio de Janeiro, 2012. [cited on December 26, 2018]. Available from: <http://bvsms.saude.gov.br/bvs/publicacoes/inca/abc_do_cancer_2ed.pdf>.

FACINA, T. Estimativa 2014 - Incidência de Câncer no Brasil. **Revista Brasileira de Cancerologia,** v.60, n.1, p.63-4,2014.

FERLAY, J. et al. Cancer incidence and mortality worldwide: sources, methods and major patterns in GLOBOCAN 2012. **International Journal of Cancer,** v.136,n.5 ,p.359-86, 2015.

FONSECA, A.J. Et al. FERREIRA MLS. Epidemiology and economic impact of cervical cancer in the state of Roraima: the SUS perspective. **Revista Brasileira de Ginecologia e Obstetricia**, v.32, n.8, p. 386-92, 2010.

GIRIANELLI, V.R et al. Disparities in cervical and breast cancer mortality in Brazil. **Revista de Saude Publica**, v. 48, n.3, p.459-67,2014.

GONZAGA, C.M.R. et al, RESENDE, A.P.M. Cervical cancer mortality trends in Brazil: 1980-2009. **Caderno de Saude Publica**, v. 29,n. 3,p.599-608, 2013.

José Alencar Gomes da Silva National Cancer Institute - INCA. **Types of cancer** [Internet]. 2014 [cited 2018 Dec 25]. Available from: http:// www2.inca.gov.br/wps/wcm/connect/tiposdecancer/site/home/colo_utero/ definiçâo.

National Cancer Institute (INCA). **Data from population-based cancer registries.** [access on 22 Dec 2018]. Available at: http://www.inca.gov.br/regpop/2003/index.asp7linkHocalizacoes. asp&ID=5.

José Alencar Gomes da Silva National Cancer Institute. **Estimate 2018: cancer incidence in Brazil**. Rio de Janeiro: INCA, 2017.

National Cancer Institute (Brazil). Estimate 2018. Incidence of Cancer in Brazil. Rio

de Janeiro: INCA, 2017. Available
at:https://www.inca.gov.br/publicacoes/livros/estimativa-2018-incidencia-de- cancer-no-brasil Accessed on:27/07/2019.

SANTOS, M. O. Estimate 2018: Cancer Incidence in Brazil. **Revista Brasileira de Cancerologia,** v.64, n.1, p.119-120, 2018.
SILVEIRA, B. L.; MAIA, R.C.B; CARVALHO, M. A. Cervical cancer: the role of nurses in the family health strategy. **FAEMA,** v. 9, n. 1, p. 348- 372, 2018.

11

CERVICAL CANCER STAGING

Aniclécio Mendes Lima

Because cervical cancer is a disease that evolves slowly, it has a high potential for prevention and cure when detected early, and this is possible because this neoplasm has a long pre-clinical phase. The staging of cervical cancer is divided into stages I, II, III and IV, and sub-classified into A or B, with IIB being seen as an advanced stage, as the tumor has metastasized beyond the uterus and invaded the parametrial region, but has not reached the pelvic wall or the lower third of the vagina, in which case there is no longer any possibility of a curative surgical approach.

The staging of cervical cancer will detail the aspects of the cancer, the degree of spread of the tumor at the time of diagnosis, i.e. whether the disease is limited only to the cervix, or whether it has radiated to organs and structures near or far from the body. Staging is determined at the time of diagnosis, and requires biopsy examination, gynecological examination, pelvic CT scan associated or not with pelvic MRI, cystoscopy, rectosigmoidoscopy and chest X-ray in order to enable accurate diagnosis and screening.

Currently, there are two systems used for staging most types of cervical cancer, the FIGO system (International Federation of Gynecology and Obstetrics) and the TNM system of the AJCC (American Joint Committee on Cancer). The FIGO system is based on the results of the clinical examination, as well as cystoscopy and proctoscopy, while the AJCC classifies cervical cancer based on 3 factors: T: Indicates the size of the primary tumor and its radiation to other areas; N: Details whether the neoplasm has spread to regional lymph nodes or whether there is evidence of metastases in transit; M: Indicates whether there is metastasis in other parts of the body (Table 1).

The TNM system uses a classification from 0 to IV to show the stage of the tumor, and the letters and numbers added after the TNM letters are for specific characteristics of the tumor. The letter T followed by a number from 0 to 4 is used to describe the tumor, including size and location. The letter N followed by numbers 0 to 3 indicates whether there has been spread to the lymph nodes and the letter M is used to indicate whether the cancer has spread to other parts of the body.

Table 01: Cervical Cancer Staging.

Internship	Description
I	Carcinoma confined to the cervix
AI	Invasive carcinoma, diagnosed only by microscopy, with a <u>maximum</u> invasion depth of < 5 m ma
IA1	Stromal invasion of up to 3 mm in depth and 7 mm or less in horizontal extension.
IA2	Cstromal invasion greater than 3 mm and up to 5 mm in depth with a horizontal extension of 7 mm or less.
IB	Clinically visible lesion confined to the cervix or microscopic lesion larger than IA2.
IB 1	Clinically visible lesion of 4 cm or less in its largest dimension.
IB 2	Clinically visible lesion over 4 cm in its largest dimension.
II	A tumor that invades beyond the uterus but does not reach the pelvic wall or the lower third of the vagina.
II A	No invasion of the parameter.
II B	Corn invasion of the parametrium.
III	Tumor that extends to the pelvic wall compromises the lower third of the vagina, or causes hydronephrosis or renal exclusion
III A	Tumor that affects the lower third of the vagina without extending to the pelvic wall.
III B	Tumor that extends to the pelvic wall, or causes hydronephrosis or renal exclusion
VAT	Tumor that invades the bladder or rectal mucosa, or extends beyond the true pelvis.
BVI	Distant metastases.

Source: FIGO, 2009.

Table 02: Surgical staging of cervical cancer.

Table 02 : Cervical cancer staging

T-PRIMARY TUMOR	
Tx	Non-Dodc tumor accessed
T0	No evidence of primary tumor
Tis	Carcinoma in situ
Tla	Invasive carcinoid tumors can only be diagnosed by microscopy; the invasion of the cervical stroma must be < 5 mm and the extension < 7 mm.
Tla1	Invasion of the strana<3mmand extension<7mm
Tla2	Invasion of the strana > 3 and < 5 mm and extension < 7 mm
Tlb	Clinical lesion confined to the uterine cavityoronricroscopic lesion greater than Пa
Tlb1	Clinical lesion < 4 cm in greatest dimension
Tlb2	Clinical lesion > 4 cm in greatest dimension
T2	Tumor invades the uterus, but not the pelvic wall or lower part of the vagina
T2a	No parametric invasion
T2a1	Clinical lesion<4cm
T2a2	Clinical lesion>4cm
T2b	Obvious invasion of parametres
T3	Tumor extends to the epididymal appendage and/or involves the lower part of the vagina and/or causes non-initiating craniorefractoriness
T3a	Bivolvement of the lower tenon of the vagina without extension to the pelvic wall
T3b	Extension to the Mcae and/or Mdroneftseourim at the bottom of the ticket
T4	Extension beyond the petve vadadara or invasion (confirmed by bicopsy) of the mucosa of the berigi or rectum. Bladder bullous edema apaiasnaopamitis that is occasionally allocated сото T4.
T4a	Invasion of the bladder mucosa or kidney Bladder bullous edema only does not allow a case to be allocated сото T4
T4b	Extension to the balcony and twelvevehicles
N-LINFONODS	
Nx	Unaccessed lymph nodes
N0	Semmetàstase paraalinfonodosieâonais
N1	Metastases to regional lymph nodes
REMOTE M-METASTASIS	
M0	No metastasis at a distance
M1	Distance metastasis

Source: AAJC, 2010.

REFERENCES

ANDRADE, J. M. et al. Screening, diagnosis and treatment of cervical carcinoma. **Projeto Diretrizes [online],** 2001.

BRAZIL. National Cancer Institute - INCA. National Cervical Cancer Control Program. Brazil, 2011c. [access on July 10, 2019].
Available at:
<http://www 1. inca.gov.br/inca/Arquivos/PROGRAMA_UTERO_internet.PDF>.

DIZ, M. P. E; DE MEDEIROS, R. B. Cancer of the uterine cervix - risk factors, prevention, diagnosis and treatment. **Revista de Medicina,** v. 88, n. 1, p. 7-15, 2009. José Alencar Gomes da Silva National Cancer Institute. **Diretrizes brasileiras para o rastreamento do câncer do colo do utero.** 2. ed. rev. ampl. atual. Rio de Janeiro: INCA, 2016. [access on August 01, 2019]. Available at:
http://www2.inca.gov.br/wps/wcm/connect/agencianoticias/site/home/noticias/2016/d iretrizes_para_rastreamento_cancer_colo_utero_consulta_publica.

José Alencar Gomes da Silva National Cancer Institute. **Brazilian guidelines for cervical cancer screening: 2016 update.** Rio de Janeiro: INCA; 2016

José Alencar Gomes da Silva National Cancer Institute. **Brazilian guidelines for cervical cancer screening: 2016 update.** Rio de Janeiro: INCA; 2016 [access on August 01, 2019]. Available at:
http://www2.inca.gov.br/wps/wcm/connect/agencianoticias/site/home/noticias/2016/d iretrizes_para_rastreamento_cancer_colo_utero_consulta_publica

SILVA, D. S. M. et al. Cervical Cancer Screening in the State of Maranhâo, Brazil. **Ciência e Saude Coletiva,** v. 19, n. 4, p. 1163-1170, 2014.

12

CERVICAL CANCER TREATMENT

Aniclécio Mendes Lima

Treatment for cervical cancer is indicated according to the FIGO staging classification based on histological type, tumor size and personal factors such as age and childbearing capacity. The main treatment options range from conservative procedures such as the removal of pre-neoplastic lesions to radical and complex treatments such as hysterectomy and/or radiotherapy. These treatments can be carried out alone or in combination, depending on the stage of the disease. In the majority of cases, surgical treatment with the removal of the uterus and the inner part of the vagina is recommended, and in young patients, if the disease is not at an advanced stage, the preservation of the ovaries is recommended.

IA1 STADIUM

The appropriate treatment for this stage is simple hysterectomy, as the risk of regional lymph node involvement is very low (1%). Oopherectomy should be dispensed with in young women and in the case of patients with genital exteriorization, the most suitable treatment is vaginal hysterectomy. In the case of patients at this stage who prioritize fertilization, the treatment indicated is conization with a scalpel or laser, as in these cases there has been no invasion of the vascular and lymphatic space. Radiotherapy-based treatment at this stage is indicated in the case of women who are unable to undergo surgery due to associated diseases, and should be treated with intracavitary irradiation.

IA2 STADIUM

The treatment indicated for women at this stage is radical hysterectomy with pelvic/para-aortic lymphadenectomy, as women present with metastases in the lymph nodes in 7% of cases and evidence of invasion of the vascular and lymphatic space in around 30%, and radiotherapy should be reserved for patients with associated diseases who are unable to undergo surgery. Oophorectomy should be avoided in premenopausal patients. In the case of patients undergoing surgical treatment who have lymph node complications, residual parametrial disease or compromised surgical margins, they should undergo external radiotherapy.

STAGE IB1

Surgical treatment with total hysterectomy with ligation of the uterine artery at the origin, parametrectomy and colpectomy of the upper 1/3 of the vagina (class III/Piver III) is the most appropriate for these patients, especially for women who are in the fertile period. radiotherapy is indicated in the case of women with associated diseases, where surgery is contraindicated. In situations where patients indicated for surgical treatment have lymph node complications, residual parametrial disease or compromised surgical margins, they should undergo external radiotherapy.

IB2 STADIUM

At this stage, the treatment indicated for women is hysterectomy including parametrectomy up to the lateral portion and removal of the cranial third of the vagina (class III/Piver III) in addition to pelvic lymphadenectomy, as the tumor is more than 4 cm in diameter and has not infiltrated the stroma of the cervix. In addition, alternative treatments for lesions at this stage include radical surgery (class III) and lymphadenectomy followed by radiotherapy if there are compromised surgical margins and parametrial invasion or metastases; external radiotherapy associated with brachytherapy; combination of radiotherapy and chemotherapy, followed or not by surgery; external radiotherapy and brachytherapy followed by radical surgery.

STADIUM IIA

Treatment with radiotherapy or radical hysterectomy is the most appropriate at this stage, and the choice of the best method will depend on the extent of the lesion in both the cervix and the vaginal wall. In cases where there has been a partial response to radiotherapy or in situations where radiotherapy cannot be carried out due to vaginal problems, surgery is more appropriate. Alternative treatments for this lesion include radical surgery (class III) with pelvic lymphadenectomy; radiotherapy (external and brachytherapy) as the sole treatment; and combinations of radiotherapy and chemotherapy followed or not by surgery.

STAGE IIB, IIIA, IIIB AND IVA

The alternatives for treating patients with advanced tumours are chemosensitization; radiotherapy alone; neoadjuvant chemotherapy followed by radiotherapy and surgery; neoadjuvant chemotherapy followed by surgery and pelvic exenteration, with the form of treatment indicated depending on each case. Chemoradiotherapy will be carried out in the same way as for stage IB2.

IVB STADIUM

At this stage, cervical cancer is an incurable disease, because the tumor cells have already invaded distant organs via the bloodstream and/or lymph. The most appropriate treatment in this situation is chemotherapy with the aim of reducing the tumors, making it possible to control the disease for as long as possible. In addition, chemotherapy can be combined with drugs that prevent the formation of blood vessels in the tumor, the most well-known of which is called bevacizumab. Another form of treatment is immunotherapy, which has been incorporated into the treatment of metastatic cervical cancer for patients who have used platinum-based chemotherapy without responding to treatment. Immunotherapy is used with the drug pembrolizumab.

REFERENCES

ANDRADE, J. M. et al. Screening, diagnosis and treatment of cervical carcinoma. **Projeto Diretrizes [online],** 2001.

BRAZIL. National Cancer Institute - INCA. National Cervical Cancer Control Program. Brazil, 2011c. [access on August 02, 2019]. Available at:
<http : //www 1. inca.gov.br/inca/Arquivos/PROGRAMA_UTERO_internet.PDF>.

CORDERO, Fernando Lopes et al. **Prognosis after treatment of cervical cancer Ib1: comparison between two surgical techniques**. 2016. Doctoral thesis.

FRIGO, L.F; ZABARDA, S. O. Cervical cancer: effects of treatment.
Revista Cinergis, v.16, n. 3, p. 164-8, 2015.

José Alencar Gomes da Silva National Cancer Institute. **Brazilian guidelines for cervical cancer screening: 2016 update.** Rio de Janeiro: INCA; 2016 [access on August 01, 2019]. Available at: http://www2.inca.gov.br/wps/wcm/connect/agencianoticias/site/home/noticias/2016/d iretrizes_para_rastreamento_cancer_colo_utero_consulta_publica.

ROCHA, S. M. M. et al. **Cytopathological profile of patients treated at Casa da Mulher and evaluation of the activity of kaurenoic acid against cervical cancer strains.** 2018. Master's thesis.

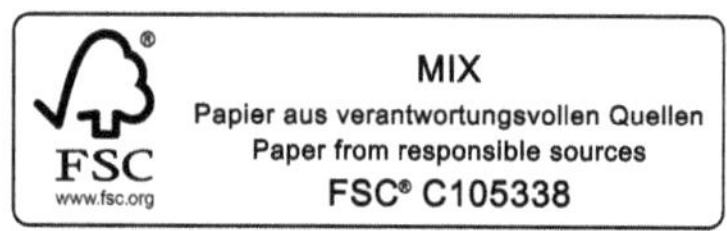

Printed by Books on Demand GmbH, Norderstedt / Germany